# Baby Shower

## Memory Book

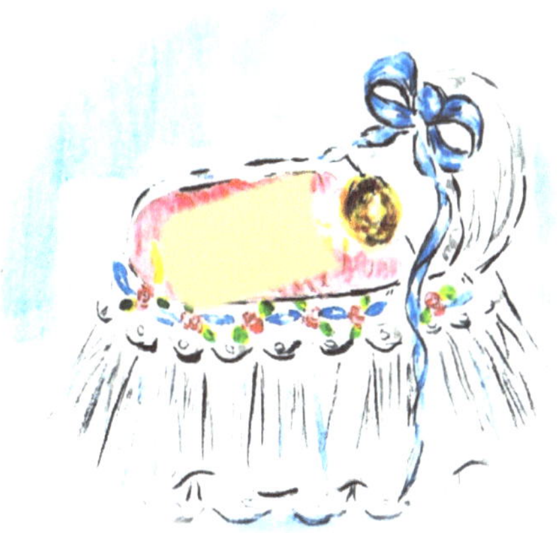

Complete organizer for baby shower
including guest and gift registry,
thank you record, and much more...

©Traditions Press, Inc. 2018

*Baby Shower Memory Book*

www.traditionspress.com

designed and illustrated by n s taylor

traditionspress@gmail.com

Lexington, SC  USA

*for Maya*

ISBN 9781546479284

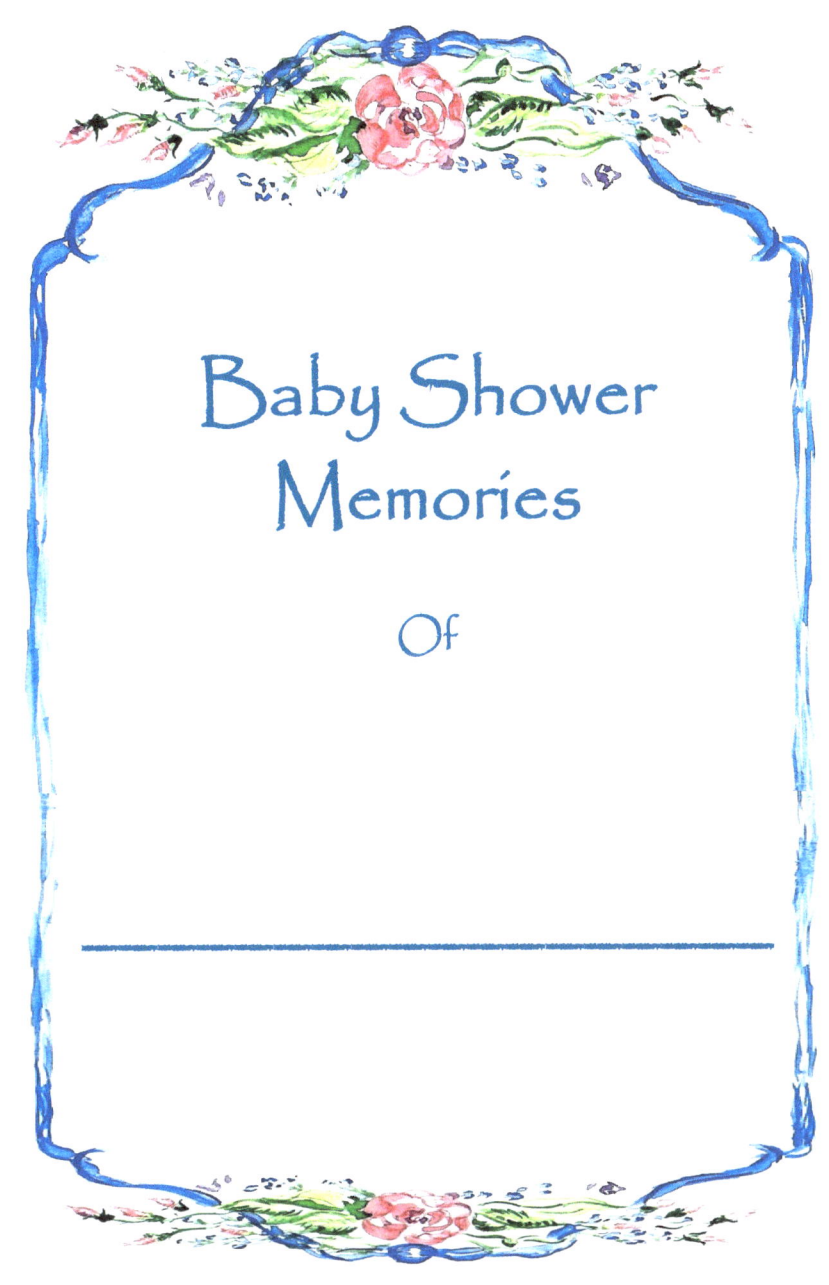

# Baby Shower
## Memories

Of

_____

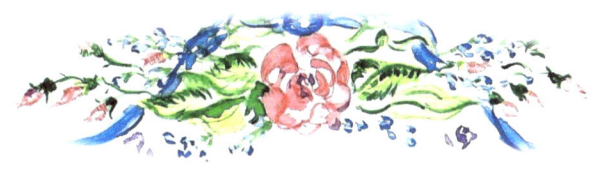

Shower photo

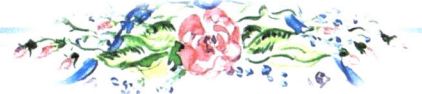

# Shower Invitation

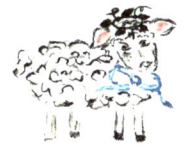 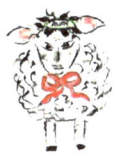 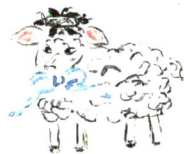

Guest Registry

By having an individual designated to greet
guests and direct them to sign the Guest Registry,
it will help insure that the mother to be has a current
and complete address to expedite
writing thank you notes.

(A thoughtful gift for the mother to be would be a couple of
boxes of thank you notes and several sheets  of the
beautiful postage stamps that are available.)

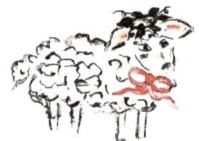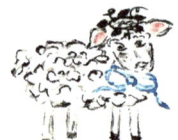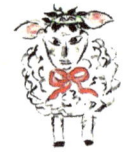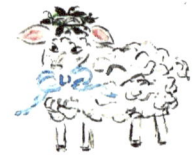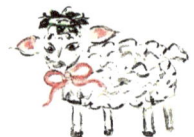

# Guests

| Name | Address | Phone | email |
|------|---------|-------|-------|
|  |  |  |  |
|  |  |  |  |
|  |  |  |  |
|  |  |  |  |
|  |  |  |  |
|  |  |  |  |
|  |  |  |  |
|  |  |  |  |
|  |  |  |  |
|  |  |  |  |

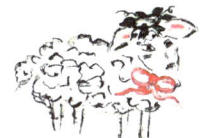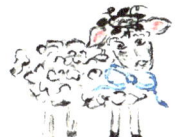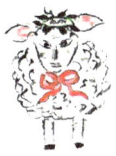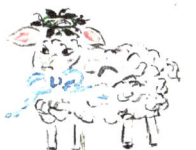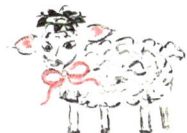

# Guests

| Name | Address | Phone | email |
|------|---------|-------|-------|
|  |  |  |  |
|  |  |  |  |
|  |  |  |  |
|  |  |  |  |
|  |  |  |  |
|  |  |  |  |
|  |  |  |  |
|  |  |  |  |
|  |  |  |  |
|  |  |  |  |

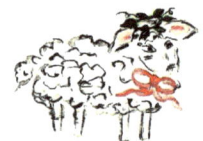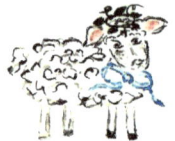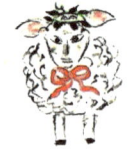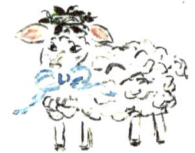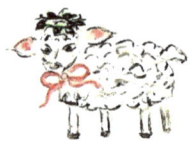

# Guests

| Name | Address | Phone | email |
|------|---------|-------|-------|
|      |         |       |       |
|      |         |       |       |
|      |         |       |       |
|      |         |       |       |
|      |         |       |       |
|      |         |       |       |
|      |         |       |       |
|      |         |       |       |
|      |         |       |       |
|      |         |       |       |

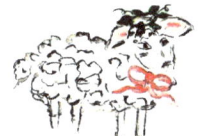 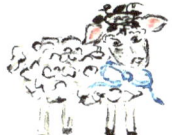 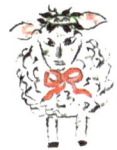 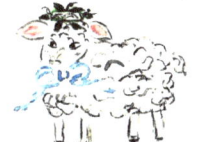 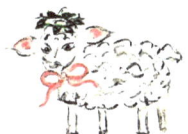

# Guests

| Name | Address | Phone | email |
|------|---------|-------|-------|
|  |  |  |  |
|  |  |  |  |
|  |  |  |  |
|  |  |  |  |
|  |  |  |  |
|  |  |  |  |
|  |  |  |  |
|  |  |  |  |
|  |  |  |  |
|  |  |  |  |

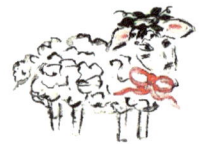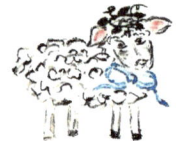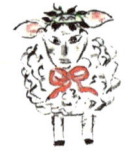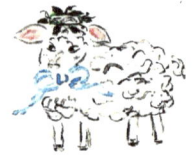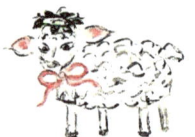

# Guests

| Name | Address | Phone | email |
| --- | --- | --- | --- |
| | | | |
| | | | |
| | | | |
| | | | |
| | | | |
| | | | |
| | | | |
| | | | |
| | | | |

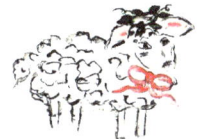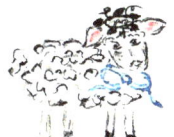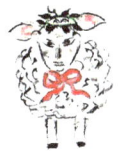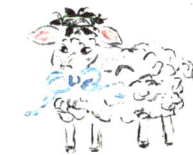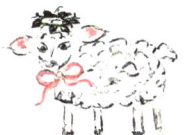

# Guests

| Name | Address | Phone | email |
|------|---------|-------|-------|
|      |         |       |       |
|      |         |       |       |
|      |         |       |       |
|      |         |       |       |
|      |         |       |       |
|      |         |       |       |
|      |         |       |       |
|      |         |       |       |
|      |         |       |       |

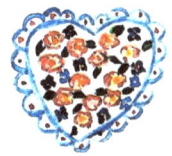 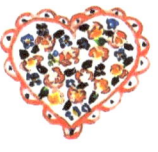 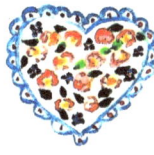

## Gift Registry

As gifts are being opened another
attendant should be recording the gift
and the person's name who brought the
gift. This is an immensely helpful
service for the mother to be. A secure
satchel or box for checks, gift cards
and other monetary gifts is good to
have available to help keep up with
financial gifts.

After the shower when it is time to start
the task of writing thank you notes the
mother to be will appreciate having
complete information available.

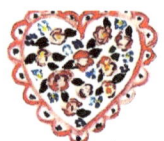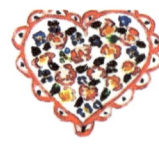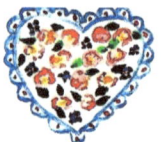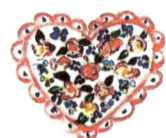

# Gift Register

| Gift | Given by | Acknowledgement Sent |
|------|----------|----------------------|
|      |          |                      |
|      |          |                      |
|      |          |                      |
|      |          |                      |
|      |          |                      |
|      |          |                      |
|      |          |                      |
|      |          |                      |
|      |          |                      |
|      |          |                      |
|      |          |                      |

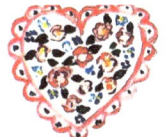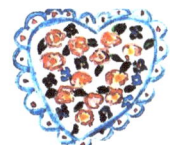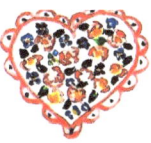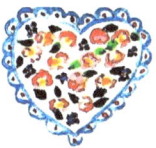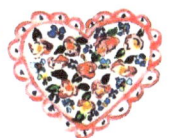

# Gift Register

| Gift | Given by | Acknowledgement Sent |
|------|----------|----------------------|
|      |          |                      |
|      |          |                      |
|      |          |                      |
|      |          |                      |
|      |          |                      |
|      |          |                      |
|      |          |                      |
|      |          |                      |
|      |          |                      |
|      |          |                      |
|      |          |                      |

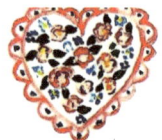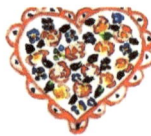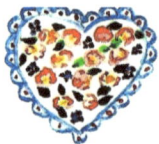

# Gift Register

| Gift | Given by | Acknowledgement Sent |
|------|----------|----------------------|
|      |          |                      |
|      |          |                      |
|      |          |                      |
|      |          |                      |
|      |          |                      |
|      |          |                      |
|      |          |                      |
|      |          |                      |
|      |          |                      |
|      |          |                      |
|      |          |                      |

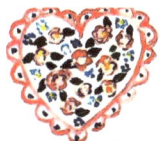 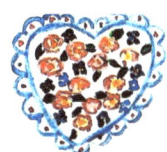 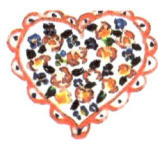 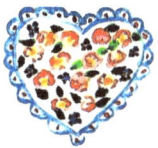 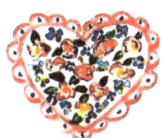

# Gift Register

| Gift | Given by | Acknowledgement Sent |
|------|----------|----------------------|
|      |          |                      |
|      |          |                      |
|      |          |                      |
|      |          |                      |
|      |          |                      |
|      |          |                      |
|      |          |                      |
|      |          |                      |
|      |          |                      |
|      |          |                      |
|      |          |                      |

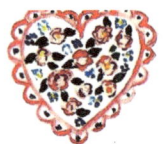 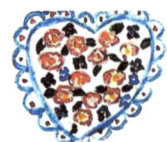 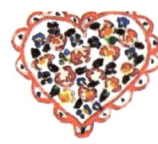 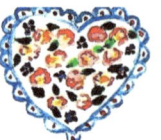 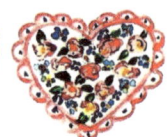

# Gift Register

| Gift | Given by | Acknowledgement Sent |
|------|----------|----------------------|
|      |          |                      |
|      |          |                      |
|      |          |                      |
|      |          |                      |
|      |          |                      |
|      |          |                      |
|      |          |                      |
|      |          |                      |
|      |          |                      |
|      |          |                      |
|      |          |                      |

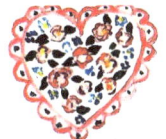 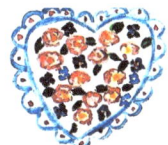 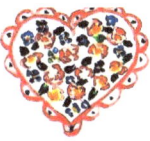 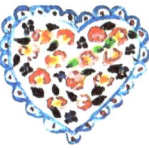 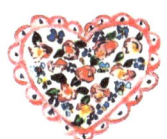

# Gift Register

| Gift | Given by | Acknowledgement Sent |
|------|----------|----------------------|
|      |          |                      |
|      |          |                      |
|      |          |                      |
|      |          |                      |
|      |          |                      |
|      |          |                      |
|      |          |                      |
|      |          |                      |
|      |          |                      |
|      |          |                      |
|      |          |                      |

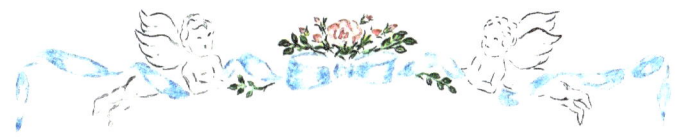

# Words of Wisdom

## for the New Mother

This section of the book may be used by guests to
write helpful sayings, quotations, scripture and
other helpful words for the new mother.
Expressions of love, encouragement and sharing
will be appreciated as they offer personal
messages preserved for the new mother
to find helpful.

(The hostess might want to include in the shower invitation
a request that attendees bring a special quote, scripture or
idea to be recorded in this book.)

# Words of Wisdom for the New Mother

Contributed by

Contributed by

Contributed by

Contributed by

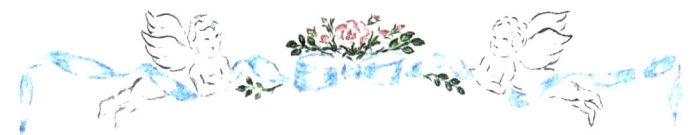

# Words of Wisdom for the New Mother

Contributed by

Contributed by

Contributed by

Contributed by

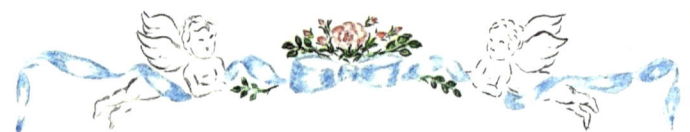

# Words of Wisdom for the New Mother

Contributed by

Contributed by

Contributed by

Contributed by

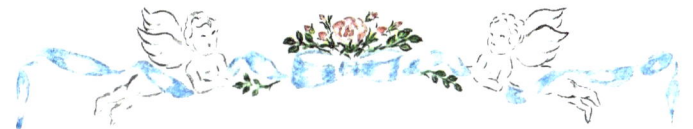

# Words of Wisdom for the New Mother

Contributed by

Contributed by

Contributed by

Contributed by

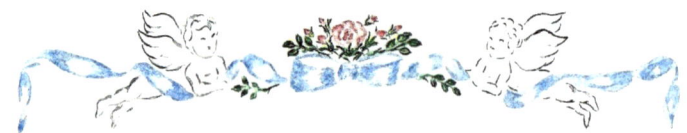

# Words of Wisdom for the New Mother

Contributed by

Contributed by

Contributed by

Contributed by

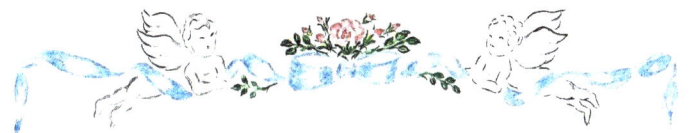

# Words of Wisdom for the New Mother

Contributed by

Contributed by

Contributed by

Contributed by

## Displaying Gifts

At the shower a table may be decorated with a suitable covering and trimmings. The gifts may be placed on the table after being opened and recorded in the gift registry. Small cards may be placed by the gifts with the name of the person giving the gift. A dinner place card is a good size for this job. Care in keeping cards with gifts should be taken when packing the gifts after the shower. There are many attractive, inexpensive large bags that are great for helping the mother to be to pack and transport her gifts.

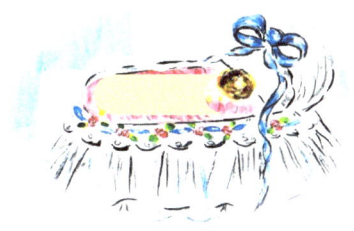

# Thank You Notes

As time and circumstances dictate, thank you
notes should be written for each gift.  This
should be done in the form of a handwritten note
within one year of receiving the gift.   Simple
note cards are sufficient; and it is good to name
the specific gift in the note.
Appreciation may be expressed about the
usefulness, matching colors and special
thoughtfulness of the gift.
Notes need not be long letters.

(Daddies can write thank you notes too!)

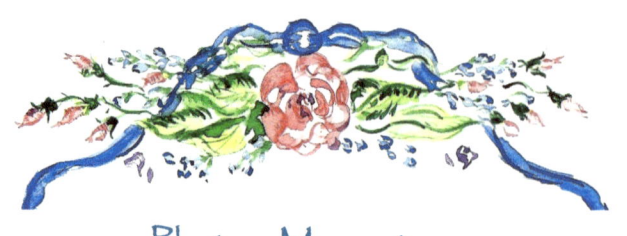

Photos, Mementos...

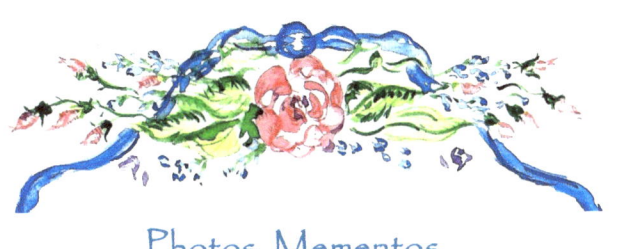

Photos, Mementos...

# Product Warranties

 Product Warranties,

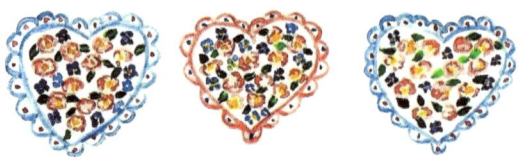

Favorite Children's Books, Movies, Websites

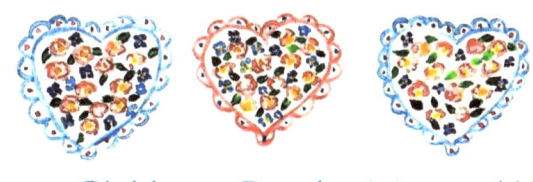

Favorite Children's Books, Movies, Websites

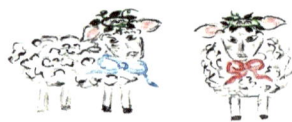

# Volunteers

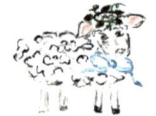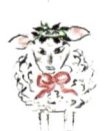

| Name/Phone/email | Errands | Babysitting | Meals date/time | Other |
|---|---|---|---|---|
|  |  |  |  |  |
|  |  |  |  |  |
|  |  |  |  |  |
|  |  |  |  |  |
|  |  |  |  |  |
|  |  |  |  |  |
|  |  |  |  |  |

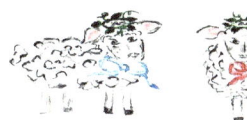 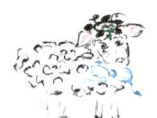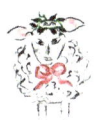

# Volunteers

| Name/Phone/email | Errands | Babysitting | Meals date/time | Other |
|---|---|---|---|---|
| | | | | |
| | | | | |
| | | | | |
| | | | | |
| | | | | |
| | | | | |
| | | | | |

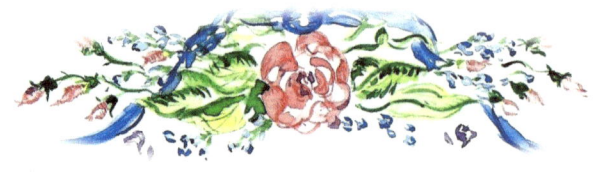

Notes

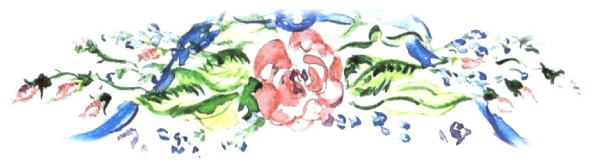

Notes